50
SMART DOGS

50
SMART DOGS

VETERINARIANS
SHARE WARM
RECOLLECTIONS

Written and Edited by Dr. Rex Puterbaugh

A BIRCH LANE PRESS BOOK
Published by Carol Publishing Group

A Birch Lane Press Book
Published by Carol Publishing Group
Birch Lane Press is a registered trademark of Carol Communications, Inc.

Editorial, sales and distribution, rights and permissions inquiries should be
addressed to Carol Publishing Group, 120 Enterprise Avenue, Secaucus, N.J. 07094.

In Canada: Canadian Manda Group, One Atlantic Avenue, Suite 105, Toronto,
Ontario, M6K 3E7

Carol Publishing Group books may be purchased in bulk at special discounts for
sales promotion, fund-raising, or educational purposes. Special editions can be
created to specifications. For details, contact Special Sales Department, Carol
Publishing Group, 120 Enterprise Avenue, Secaucus, N.J. 07094.

Manufactured in the United States of America
10 9 8 7 6 5 4 3 2 1

Library of Congress Cataloging-in-Publication Data

50 smart dogs: veterinarians share warm recollection/edited by Rex
    Puterbaugh.
        p.   cm.
    "A Birch Lane Press book."
    ISBN 1–55972–476–5 (hc)
    1. Dogs—United States—Anecdotes.   2. Veterinarians—United
States—Anecdotes. I. Puterbaugh, Rex.
SF426.2.A153   1998
636.7—dc21   98–19095
                                                                CIP

*I dedicate this book to my four sons,
Bill, Jim, Geoff, and Kip and to their families—
and in memory of my wife, Elaine.
My sons have given me 5 percent worry and
95 percent great pleasure and pride.*

CONTENTS

Acknowledgments   9
Preface   11
Introduction   15

My Own Experiences   *23*
Veterinarian Yarns   *31*
Retrieval Tales   *47*
Courageous Dogs   *65*
Smart Dogs   *77*
Extraordinary Escapes   *87*
Family Dogs   *91*
Hightailing to the Hospital   *105*
A Nose for Direction   *123*
Memorable Tales   *129*

Acknowledgments

There are many people I have to thank for the help they have given me.

First, I thank all the people who sent in their letters. It was difficult to pick out the best, and I'm sure I passed up some that could have been used.

I would like to thank my four sons and Dr. Mil Custer, who all gave constructive criticism, and many others who made helpful suggestions.

I also want to thank the editor and producer of the book "The Prairie Practitioner," for letting me use some of the articles in this book. (It is available from SDVMA, Box 2175, South Dakota State University, Brooking, South Dakota 57077.)

I want to thank Tom Estes, the artist, who did such fine work with the cartoons and caricatures. I also want to thank my step-daughter, Nancy Benson, who checked the stories and gave very good advice, and a very special thanks to my daughter-in-law, Candy Puterbaugh. She spent many hours recommending changes and improvements, and suggesting titles and cartoons for many of the stories.

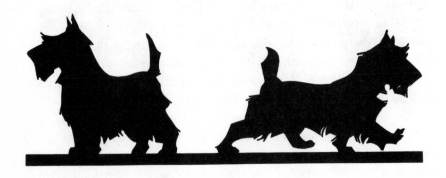

PREFACE

If someone says the world has gone to the dogs, that may bode well for the world. Dogs have a pretty good place in it. They have carved themselves a nice niche next to their masters and it's likely to stay that way. The dog has been man's best friend at least since the Stone Age, when he kept his caveman company.

History is full of evidence of man's love for his dog...and vice-versa. The ancient Egyptians made dogs into a god. And when a pet dog died, members of an Egyptian family would cut off their hair in mourning.

Buried under lava in 79 A.D., the city of Pompeii was uncovered in the eighteenth century. Across the skeleton of a little girl, as if trying to protect her, was the skeleton of a dog. And on the dog's collar was an inscription praising him for once saving his master's life from a wolf.

It was thought by many that dogs originated from wolves, jackals, and coyotes. Recent use of DNA has shown that the wolf was probably the one and only ancestor of the dog. There is good evidence that wolves were in the process of becoming domesticated 135,000 years ago. We believe that dogs were domesticated at least 14,000 years ago. At that time, humans were hunters and gatherers, and the dog probably helped with the hunting.

About ten thousand years ago, humans learned how to plant and grow food, so they became farmers instead of hunters. The dog was not needed as much to hunt as to guard the farmer's property.

All this time, as humans were becoming more intelligent, so were the dogs. From about 500 B.C. to 500 A.D., in Roman times, dogs were being bred for special purposes (hunting, guarding, herding, etc.), but the proliferation of the modern breeds didn't start until the thirteenth century.

Today there are 132 breeds of dogs in all shapes and sizes. The one thing we can agree on about dogs is that, like humans, they are all different. A St. Bernard can weigh three hundred pounds to a Chihuahua's one-and-a-half pounds. On the run, a pointer can tell if a quail, yards away, is wounded or dead, while a Pekingese probably can't tell a pig from a possum a yard away.

Dogs also come with different brains. During my forty

years as a veterinarian, I have seen and heard of some amazing feats of intelligence from this animal who is seemingly most content at his master's feet.

As you may have noted, there are always articles in the newspaper or on television of heroic and intelligent feats dogs have accomplished. I have read about dogs waking their masters in the middle of the night because the house was on fire. There was a recent article about a small child who was choking, and the dog barked to alert an adult and save the child's life. There is also the story about an elderly man who was fly fishing, slipped on a rock, fell, and was knocked unconscious. When he awoke, he was on dry land. His dog pulled him out of the water and prevented him from drowning.

You may have heard that certain dogs can be trained to alert an epileptic before he has a seizure. No one knows for certain how they can tell, but it is thought by some that the person might give off an odor detectable only by the dog. It is a well-known fact that a dog's sense of smell is a hundred times stronger than a human's. Such evidence only reinforces the fact that dogs are very special animals.

Always having had an interest in intelligent dogs—and noting that most every professional that I've met at veterinarian conferences and meetings has an interesting story to tell or had a memorable medical event occur—I decided to write this book.

To gather data on this, I sent over five thousand letters to those in the veterinary profession. I have also included my own experiences, as well as stories that I've heard over the years. I hope you enjoy them as much as I have.

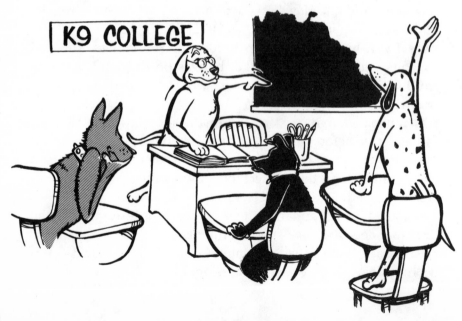

INTRODUCTION

I began the practice of veterinary medicine in 1940 in suburban Chicago while working with an older, established veterinarian. Most young vets work with an older vet for a time— a kind of internship—learning all the hands-on medical applications they didn't learn in college. I was very fortunate to work with this particular veterinarian, as he was a good teacher. I more or less ran his small-animal hospital while he and another young vet ran the large animal practice. I would fill in for them at times, and they for me.

After about a year, I learned of a practice for sale in Indiana. I borrowed some money and bought the practice (and the house and office space that went with it) for $8,000. There I did a mixed practice, much like James Herriot did in his *All Creatures Great and Small* book series. While Herriot's experiences and mine were often quite similar, it seemed to me that whenever he had a case he really cared about, the patient lived.

In my case, many of the ones I cared about and worked hardest to save often died.

During World War II, I became extremely busy, starting my day at 5:30 A.M. most days, and doing small-animal work in the evening. It was hard, tiring work. My wife was taking care of our four boys and the office—sometimes with additional help, but mostly alone, since help during this time was hard to find. After the war, we had to make a decision whether to buy another house, build an animal hospital on the edge of town, and hire another veterinarian, or buy an animal hospital in another area. I decided that if I were ever going to make a change, this was the time to do it. We decided to sell and move to California.

I started advertising for a small-animal hospital. We had heard about the beautiful seaside village of La Jolla, which at that time was tiny—no stoplights, very little traffic, good schools, excellent weather, and very few people who locked their doors. It was the ideal place to raise four sons.

We soon found ourselves in La Jolla, visiting the site where a vet was building a new animal hospital. We bought it after six months of dickering; I sold my own practice, and took the California State Board exams. We named it the La Jolla

Veterinary Hospital. It bears the same name today after nearly fifty years, and is run by four extremely capable veterinarians.

It was in La Jolla that I became interested in intelligent dogs, mostly because of one litter of poodles and their owner. She gave these pups—four black and three honey colored—to some of her friends, and then she and their new owners all bragged about the smart things these dogs could do. I was fortunate enough to be the caretaker of most of the litter.

One gentleman told me that when he came home from work, he always went to the closet, took off his shoes, and put on slippers. One day when he came home, his litterpick ran to the closet and came back with a slipper, then ran back and brought another one. Once the gentleman had removed his shoes to put on the offered slippers, his dog proceeded to take the removed shoes to the closet. From that day on, the dog performed this task, and also brought in the newspaper without being told.

Another owner told me about her female poodle, Liz. The woman's husband was a stockbroker and always arose at 6:00 every morning, and she would fix breakfast while her husband took Liz out for a short walk. After Liz did her morning business, he would reward her with a dog treat. Liz seemed to be able to differentiate between weekdays and weekends, but holidays were another matter entirely. One Monday morning, a holiday, a little after 6:00, Liz came into the bedroom and barked at him. "What's wrong with her?" he complained. "I guess she doesn't know it's a holiday," his wife replied. This 6 A.M. wakeup reminder was repeated on a weekday holiday as well.

When one dog's master became ill and was driven a mile and a half away to a clinic, his dog came along for the ride. When it turned out that the master had to stay overnight, the dog was brought home. The next morning, however, the dog was missing, and the family frantically began looking for her everywhere, until they got a call from the clinic; the dog was there. He had climbed up the fire escape from the rear of the clinic and had been found scratching on the outside of his master's door. I didn't believe this, so I called the clinic and they confirmed it.

A man watched his friend playing poker with his dog. "That must be a very smart dog to be able to play poker," he remarked.

"Oh, he's not so smart," the friend answered. "Every time he gets a good hand, he wags his tail."

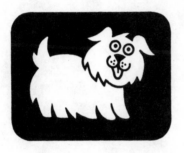

50
SMART DOGS

My Own Experiences

After a veterinary practice of forty years, I've met a good number of smart dogs. Here are a few tales of my own:

My client's wonderful Labrador had puppies. I told him I wanted a pup, and when the litter was about seven weeks old, I went over to take my pick. I used the old trick of putting an alarm clock in with the pups. The first one to check it out after it rang was generally the one to take. One male turned around immediately, went over to the clock, and looked curiously at it. He was the one for me. My boys named him Merlin.

Merlin was a wonderful pet. Over the years, our household had fish, three cats, three dogs, a chinchilla, a king snake, hamsters, a cockatoo, and a mouse. But in all the years, none compared with Merlin.

We had a large, fenced backyard, but Merlin turned out to be a great escape artist. Of course, with four boys, I have always suspected that Merlin might have had a little help—sometimes accidental, sometimes not—but as soon as the boys got home from school, Merlin would always return home.

One time, when we had to go out of town, we boarded Merlin at the animal hospital. Because he was such a magician, we had to leave specific directions for wiring his cage door shut. Of course someone goofed, and the kennel man heard all the dogs barking. Upon investigation, he found that not only had Merlin let himself out but had opened up five other dog runs. After the kennel man returned all the dogs to their appropriate runs, Merlin remained missing. Finally, he was found in the surgery, shacked up with a female Irish setter. Luckily, she was not in heat.

Two months after our youngest son went to college, Merlin died. We have always wondered: old age or a broken heart?

All in a Day's Work

One day, George, my employer, a gruff yet fair man, walked in on me as I was treating a dog. "Isn't that Joey Johnson?" he asked, pointing to the dog. I answered affirmatively that it was. "Why do you have him muzzled?" George asked. "He wouldn't bite a fly." And he proceeded to take off the muzzle before I could stop him. Wouldn't you know it, Joey turned around and bit him. There was a stream of obscenities as the boss quickly pulled his arm back and left to bandage it.

Despite the appearance, however, George was a real animal lover. He had a pet Welsh terrier, Bonny, and a cat. Sometimes, when the hospital was quiet, he would get in his big overstuffed chair and take a nap with Bonny and the cat beside him.

A client had two German shepherds, one male and one female. The male was an accomplished escape artist; no leash could keep him. At the veterinary hospital in La Jolla, we kept our leashes in a small alcove off the main hallway. One day, I heard a noise there. Investigating, I found that not only had our male German shepherd escaped from his run and shaken his leash off; he was also attempting to shake off his sister's leash.

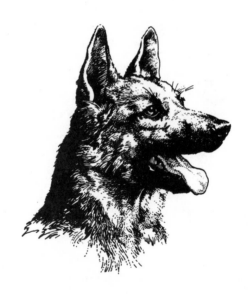

The Call of Nature

One woman told me she was in her kitchen one morning when her German shepherd gently put his jaw over her hand and tried to pull her. When she told him to stop, he started pulling on her dress. Finally, she got the idea that he wanted her to follow him. He led her out the back door and headed for the alley, looking back all the time to make sure she was coming behind. They finally ended up at a garage door all the way down the alley, where the dog started scratching on the door. At this time, a lady came out of the neighboring house and asked what was going on. The lady said, "There's nothing wrong here. The only thing in my garage is my dalmatian in heat!"

Good Directions

One man told me about his Labrador-whippet cross named Bud. One day, he, his wife, and Bud took a trip from their home in upper New York state to Manhattan to visit his brother who lived on the Upper East Side, a populous area. They stayed the day. Several months later, they again drove to Manhattan to take some courses downtown at New York University. Bud was left in the car with the door unlocked, but with an on-site attendant. When they returned after class, Bud was gone.

The couple was devastated. They searched the neighborhood and finally placed an ad in the newspapers, but remember that New York is one Big Apple. No word of Bud came.

Luckily, about ten days after losing Bud, they received a call asking if they were missing a black dog. Excited, they immediately drove to the address of the caller who turned out to live on the same street as the owner's brother. The gentleman who called them said he observed Bud roaming the neighborhood for several days. Bud had a short rope on his collar that appeared to have been chewed off, and the gentleman was able to grasp the rope and read the identification.

After exuberant thanks, the couple were amazed that Bud could find his way to a neighborhood he'd only visited once before.

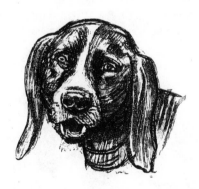

Smart Collie

A collie, owned by a colleague's client, was a Lassie fan. Whenever the TV show would come on, the collie would become very excited. During one particular episode, she almost went berserk, barking and running around uncontrollably. When the owner looked up to the television screen, she saw that a mountain lion was about to pounce on Lassie. The collie, the veterinarian said with glee, was warning Lassie to get out of there.

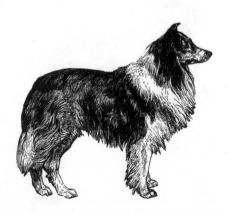

Veterinarian Yarns

Following are stories from across the country, submitted by veterinarians who have met many remarkable dogs—and people—in their time. Most of the stories will give you a chuckle or touch your heart with kindness.

Off to the Races

Reprinted with permission from *The Prairie Practitioners*

Dachshund dogs are prone to develop back problems due to their very long bodies, and can become paralyzed in their rear legs. Many veterinarians gave up on them and sent them to us at the veterinary college. Some we could help by surgery and

31

other treatments, but many had so much damage to the spinal cord that nothing could be done.

Someone developed a small wheeled cart that strapped onto the dog's rear end so it could get around. It was a sort of wheelchair for dachshunds. At one time, we had four of the wheelchair dogs at the small-animal clinic. In the evening, when all the professors were gone, we had them race in a long, wide hallway.

They were all named, and I had them all handicapped (pardon the pun). Slow Moe was the slowest and Greased Lightning was the fastest. Sea Biscuit and Silver Bullet were somewhere in the middle. I discovered that if we placed Greased Lightning three feet behind the starting line, and Slow Moe two feet in front of it, it made for a nice tight race. They were all rewarded at the finish line with a piece of dog candy or a milk bone. The winner would get double portions.

The dogs came to love the races. I'm sure it was the high point of their day. However, the powers that be heard about them and made us stop.

I miss the races because they helped defray some of my college expenses. The rest of the students missed them because they were a lot of fun, and I think that the dogs missed them as much as—or more than—we did.

Wily Yvette

Submitted by Dr. Leonard Witt, Fremont, Nebraska

Three poodles—half toy and half miniature—came to our hospital. We had to hand raise and bottle feed the three poodles for several weeks. Everyone took an immediate liking to the female and we named her Yvette.

Right away you could see how wily she was. She quickly had the two males hoodwinked when feeding time came around. When we fed the three of them, she would take some food out of the dish and act like it was the greatest tidbit in the world. Curious and competitive, the males would come over to take it away, and while they were fighting each other over it, she would consume the larger portion.

Her wiliness grew as she became older. When my wife or I wanted to take her for a walk, Yvette would become very excited when it was mentioned. So we soon started to spell it. After the fourth time she heard W-A-L-K, she caught on and would always head for her leash.

Smell the Roses

Submitted by J. Fred Smithcors, DVM, Santa Barbara, California

For seventeen years, my wife and I enjoyed the playfulness and companionship of our part-miniature dachshund, Gretel. For most of this time, Gretel slept in the powder room, and promptly at 7:30 each morning she would yip once to be let out. Upon being let out the back door, she would run across the lawn and stop at the head of the garden path to sniff the dwarf roses, then amble some 40 or 50 yards down the path, stopping frequently to investigate other flowers and plants. After fifteen or twenty minutes, Gretel would race back to the door as if to make certain she would see me before I left for work.

When she was about sixteen, Gretel developed congestive heart failure and had to be helped down and back up the steps for her morning routine, which never varied except for progressively shortening her walk and slowing her pace back to the door as her condition worsened. One morning, she yipped long before daylight, at 2:30. I was so slow that she impatiently scratched at the door. Her condition had obviously deteriorated considerably, and so I carried her out to the garden, where she smelled the roses briefly and then looked up at me as if to indicate she was satisfied. I carried her back,

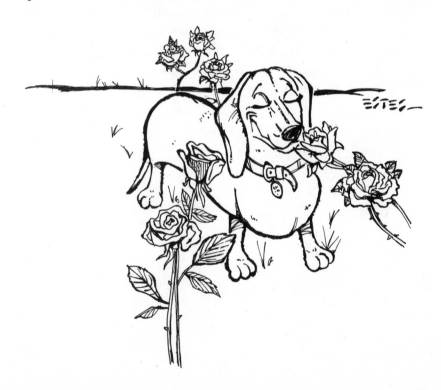

and she licked my hand as I put her in her bed. Later we missed her customary yip at wake-up time, and upon investigation found she had died.

Whether this change in Gretel's routine was mere chance, or an instance of canine prescience, we'll never know. But later I wished I had been prescient enough to have plucked a rose that early morning for her to smell in bed.

Fittingly, we buried her in the rose garden.

Too Much Discipline?

Submitted by Dr. H. W. Knirk, Lansing, Michigan

A lady brought a very sick dog with a high temperature to my clinic. She wanted the dog hospitalized until it was completely well. The dog ultimately responded well to treatment, and was playful and happy to see us, wagging its tail. However, it refused to eat. We tempted it with a smorgasbord of foods: meats, tidbits from our own meals, dog foods and the like. Still no response.

After several days, I called the owner, trying to encourage her to take her pet home. Maybe then it would eat for her. She refused, saying, "No, I want the dog to be normal." She called a few moments later and cautiously asked if I had said *okay* after I offered the food. She explained that her family was afraid someone might poison the dog, so they had trained him not to eat until he heard that command.

I went back to the dog's cage, put down several kinds of food, and said "Okay." The dog devoured everything. I returned to the phone and demanded that the woman come get her dog. It had starved itself for four days because of its discipline.

There are more than
fifty-five million dogs
in the United States.

Trail Etiquette

Submitted by Jessica Breinholt, Coalville, Utah

There are only a few choice places in northern Utah where conditions are suited to the running of sled dogs, and very often they are perfect for snowmobilers as well. And so we share them, attempting to follow etiquette and smiling politely at the curious stares we receive, as we unload dogs and prepare sleds. The snowmobilers, though, tend to neglect etiquette, forgetting that the dogs are living beings quite capable of fear and discomfort at the growling, belching machines that swarm around them.

On a cold, sunny morning in February, we prepare to run. The dogs stand on short chains hooked to a picket line that extends from the side of the truck, six Siberian huskies of varying color and size. There are four standing in the long, narrow aisle created by the trail, including Tigger. He is a large grey and white male with one brown eye and the other one pale blue. This gives him a sort of chaotic, half-crazed expression that never fails to catch the eye of the curious.

Today we are busy harnessing the dogs, and do not notice the approach of three snowmobiles until they come to a rumbling halt directly beside us. Their riders dismount and walk away, leaving the machines running. The dogs eye them nervously, pressing closer to the truck and fidgeting on their chains. Tigger is placed in the lead position, accompanied by a small white female, and we take off just as the snowmobilers return.

The silence of the forest and the soft sound of the dogs' breath is quietly comforting after the roaring din of the snow machines, and we run without speaking, listening to the crunch of paws, two on snow and the faint whisk of sled runners moving down the trail. The dogs hear it before we do, and it is only when they begin darting occasional, doubtful glances over their shoulders that we stop breathing to really listen. After a moment, we can hear it, too, the faint sharp whine of artificial transportation. We feel the dogs slowing, too distracted by the growing noise to concentrate on running. We speak to them, encouraging them to ignore the sounds and move on. It is, as usual, a futile effort.

The snowmobiles appear a few moments later, careening toward the team with no apparent intention of slowing down. They flash past, engines screaming, cutting so close to the team that Tigger trips over the little female next to him in his effort to get out of the way. "Slow down!" we yell, as they disappear up the narrow trail in a cloud of snow and exhaust. As the noise dies away, the dogs pick up speed, settling back into a light, quick trot. We hear voices as we round a wide corner, and see ahead of us the abandoned hulk of three snowmobiles. They are parked side by side across the trail, taking nearly all of its frugal width.

It becomes immediately apparent that we cannot get both dogs and sled past the snowmobiles intact; there simply isn't enough room. We look around for the riders, eventually seeing the same men who had first left their machines running next to the truck, standing in the deep snow several feet off the trail. They stand with their backs to us, speaking loudly, pointing, and gesturing across the small canyon through which the trail runs. One turns to glance over his shoulder and, seeing us, waves and says, "We'll be there in a minute." He turns back to his colleagues. The dogs begin to look around restlessly, getting bored. The leaders are trained to stand and hold the team when we stop; they can bark, jump in place, and even eat snow, but they cannot move to the sides of the trail for any reason. This holds especially true for the males, for fear they might lead the team off in search of some pine tree trunk upon which to raise a leg. Tigger and his partner stand solidly at the front of the team, staring at us over the heads of the other dogs, utterly annoyed at the delay.

After several minutes, the three men tramp back onto the trail. They are met by the eager barks and leaping bodies of a sled dog team that has waited too long. The men smile blandly as they climb onto their machines, start them in a puff of exhaust, and maneuver just far enough so that we might be able to squeeze past. After such a lengthy wait, we expect the team to bolt when the brake is released, but an intimidated silence has descended over the dogs at the resurrection of the snowmobiles. We prepare to thank them grudgingly as the team inches past, but pause when we see Tigger sidle close to the pointed nose of one machine, give it a disdainful sniff as he glances up at its rider, and calmly lift his leg. A strained silence follows, broken by the cheerful tap of liquid on plastic. We can only grin, waving, as good trail etiquette dictates, when the team finally trots away.

Bath Time

Submitted by Barbara A. Huffman, Urbana, Illinois

On April 19, 1996, several tornadoes touched down near our home in St. Joseph, Illinois. My fifteen-year-old daughter, Amanda, was home alone. I called her from work to tell her to go down to the basement. She hated the thought of going into the basement by herself, as the power had gone out. Amanda decided to call our two dogs in. One dog, Honey, is a terrier/pit bull mix and the other, Lucky, is a terrier/beagle mix. Honey went right downstairs to the basement with her, but as hard as she tried, Amanda could not get Lucky to go with her.

After the storm passed, Amanda went upstairs looking for Lucky. She looked around a while and finally found Lucky in the perfect place—the bathtub. Now, Lucky is a good dog but she HATES baths. We decided that she must have watched all the shows that tell you to go to the safest place in the house. She is one smart dog!

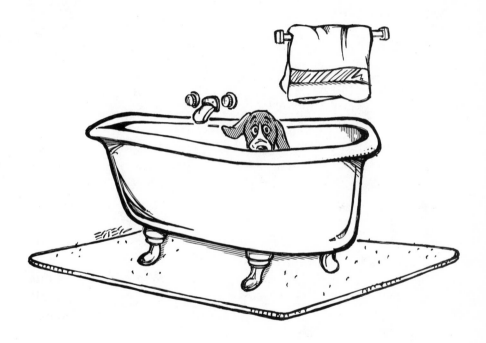

Retrieval Tales

Abby Gets a Chance to Show Off Her Tricks

Submitted by Dr. Robert Laurence, Palm Beach Gardens, Florida.
Used by permission of the *Palm Beach Post*

One plus three.

"Woof, woof, woof, woof," barked Abby, her long black and white tail wagging furiously.

Five minus three.

"Woof, woof," Abby replied, eyeing the beer bottle in Jimmy Smith's hands and hoping for a more interesting game.

The three-year-old mixed breed, once destined for the dog pound, jumped and wagged and panted with excitement as

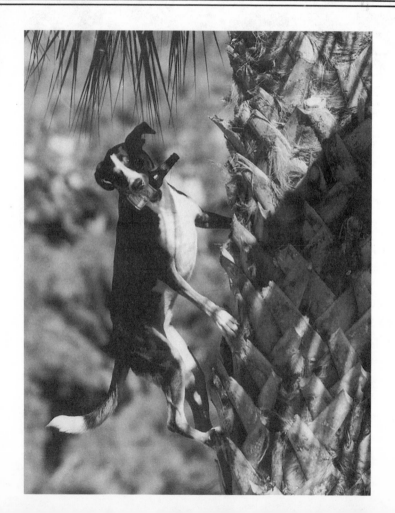

Smith took a Budweiser bottle and wedged it in the bark of a palm tree about fifteen feet off the ground.

"Get the bottle!" Smith urged. Abby happily obliged—leaping up the tree, scrabbling for paw holds until she snagged the long-necked bottle in her teeth and proudly delivered it to Smith.

That's not all. She can shinny up pine trees, climb ladders, and open refrigerator doors. She even pops the metal bottle cap off with her teeth.

Smith adopted Abby about two years ago when a friend said he planned to take her to the animal shelter. (Abby had a penchant for digging holes and other misdeeds.)

But Smith saw something else in the black, white, and tan pooch that might be part German shepherd and part Labrador retriever. He recognized the dog's cleverness.

One day, Smith was enjoying a cold beer after work and tucked it in a tree for a moment.

Abby went and got it.

After that, Abby grew so fond of retrieving, Smith found he could put a bottle just about anywhere and Abby would find it.

A Rock Hound

Submitted by Dr. Busch, Chokio, Minnesota

After treating an animal on a farm near Artichoke Lake, I stood with the farmer talking by the lake.

He said, "I'll bet you a dollar if I throw a rock out there, about thirty feet out, my Labrador will retrieve it." The lake was very shallow at that end, about two-feet deep, and I knew this was going to be the easiest dollar I'd make that day. He picked up an unusual shaped rock, about the size of a small orange, breathed on it, and threw it a good thirty feet into the lake. He said, "Bo, go get it." The dog charged out and brought the identical rock back. I couldn't believe it.

A few days later, I drove by the farm and asked if his dog could fetch the rock again. He wanted to know if I wanted to bet on it. I told him, "No, but I would like to see if the dog could do it again," which he promptly did.

I told a friend of mine about it. He said, "That's impossible." So I took him out to the farm. He watched in amazement when the dog retrieved the rock. He said, "The only way I could have found that rock was to have the lake drained."

Dog of Many Talents

Submitted by Dr. W. P. Berner, San Rafael, California

A loving wife wanted to honor her husband's upcoming birthday with a special gift. He was an avid hunter and longed for a good hunting dog. She decided to purchase a trained dog, provided there was a trial run before the purchase. The seller also agreed that the husband could bring along a couple of buddies on a hunting trip.

When the group arrived at the farm to try out the selected dog, they were told there were pheasants in the fields, and if they wanted to try the dog on quail, there were some in the creek by the willow trees.

The pheasant hunt went perfectly. Each hunter got his birds because of the exactness of the dog's pointing and retrieving. They agreed to try the quail area, and there, too, were dramatically good results on the part of dog and men. As they sat and contemplated this ideal hunt, one of the fellows absentmindedly broke off a long willow branch. When he did that, the dog saw it and raced off to the farmhouse. When the hunting party reached the farmhouse, they queried the farmer about beating the dog with a willow branch. "Oh, no," said the farmer. "I would never in the world try to train a dog by beating." Then he said, "I saw the dog come running back. He went straight to the garden area. He thought you fellows wanted to go fishing. He's back there now, digging up the garden so you can get some fishing worms. After all, he saw your long willow and it looked like my fishing pole."

The wife bought the dog and her husband raved for years about this marvelous animal, and that he was the perfect gift.

No Ducks for Dude

Submitted by R. G. MacKintosh, DVM, Yakima, Washington

An old friend invited me to a duck-hunting club because I had taken care of his Labrador retriever, Dude. This big and overweight dog lay on the floor of the duck blind on his gunny sack, and peered out of a hole facing the pond where the wooden decoys floated gently. The hiss of wings signaled approaching birds. This told me and Dude to be ready. I stood and fired twice as the mallards powered in. They flared up and away, but Dude plunged into the icy water for his retrieve. However, there were no ducks. I am not the world's best wing shot. I gestured to the dog to wait, and it wasn't long until the ducks returned. BANG! BANG! As the ducks flew away I noticed that the dog had gone out of his hole in the blind and stood belly-deep in the water. No plunging retrieve this time; just an observation. Dude looked back at me, walked back into his bed, shook himself, and lay down. I apologized to old Dude, and promised, "next time."

Twenty minutes later, he looked up at me—when we heard

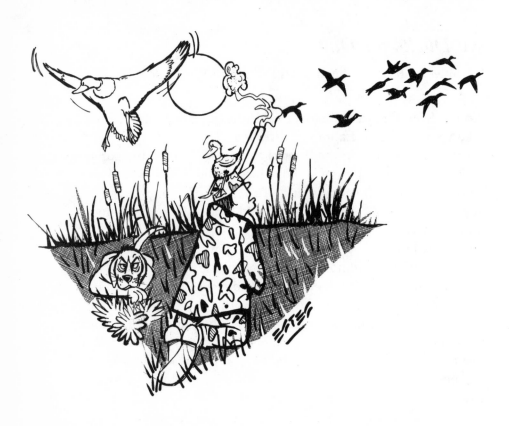

the sound of wings. I fired twice. Dude arose and went to his little doorway, looked out, and then lay back down once more. When he looked at me this time, I felt quite humble.

Again I fired and missed. You'd think I would have learned. Dude had. He opened his eyes from his nap, looked at me, turned over, and went back to sleep.

Do you think dogs can't think? They don't even need to talk.

Portia and the Giant Fish

Submitted by Coriane Gloger, Chicago, Illinois

Dr. Bruno named a fine young butterscotch pup Portia and made her part of the Bruno family, which included another female dog named Nessa. Dr. Bruno had rescued Nessa as a pup from the rough Chicago streets and, under his care, Nessa had recovered and even went on to fame.

Nessa had actually learned to water ski! She did it regularly on a special pair of children's skis lashed together and carpeted, and had been the subject of front-page coverage in the Chicago papers. Nessa was always the center of attention when Dr. Bruno and the dogs made an outing along the shore of the lake.

Was Portia jealous of all the attention lavished on Nessa?

Well, one Friday when the water was choppy, Dr. Bruno, Nessa, and Portia were unable to go for a swim in their usual spot, so they wandered on toward the harbor. They drew up above a rocky inlet and discovered that a few young fishermen and sailors had managed to cut off a huge fish and trap it in the inlet, and were amusing themselves trying to catch it. The fish was enormous, at least twenty pounds in weight and a yard in length.

Suddenly, to everyone's amazement, Portia leapt from the rocks above the inlet and dove nine feet straight into the water. Everyone stopped and turned to gaze in astonishment at the bubbles in the water. Where was Portia? In the next instant, the dog surfaced with the fish! Portia held the giant fish helpless between her legs, straddling the huge thing and trying to figure out what to do next. She tried to maneuver the fish to shore, but she and the fish were the same size. Finally Dr. Bruno and a couple of the sailors decided to rescue Portia and spare the fish.

With difficulty, Portia was separated from her prize and dragged back up the rocks overlooking the inlet. At this point, Portia leapt again! She dove right back into the lake and caught the poor giant fish all over again, and had to be removed yet another time from her helpless fishy victim.

By now, everyone but the fisher dog, Portia, was ready to move on to some new adventure. Dr. Bruno and his two dogs turned north to their swimming spot, but Portia could be seen looking in the direction of her relinquished prize. As the day wore on there was still great pride in the eyes and the carriage of the butterscotch dog, and surely there was envy in the eyes of her famous sister, Nessa.

An Excellent Retriever

Submitted by Dr. Benjamin Sann, Tucson, Arizona

David, our weimaraner, had been a great retriever since he was a puppy. We found this out one summer day when we took him to a pond deep enough to swim in. I threw a stick into the water and David hesitated at first, but then jumped in and realized he could swim. A look of amazement came over his face and, once ashore, he was ready to go back in and swim. Whenever we passed a body of water after that, David would start to bark, wagging his tail, telling me "Let's stop! I want to go swimming!"

David loved to play ball with me on the hill behind my old house. Naturally, I would tire of the game a lot sooner than he would. I figured that if I could just throw that ball up the hill long enough, David would get tired and want to quit. One day, I threw the ball nonstop, and it was not long before David retrieved the ball, came back down the hill, and ran right by me and into the house. No more for him that day!

On the Quail's Trail

Submitted by Dr. L. C. Thompson, Vidalia, Georgia

My field trial bird dogs have placed over three hundred times in twenty-four championships. But I've never seen one that even comes close to "Hayride Robert Thompson," also known as Bob.

I could put a marble in a bucket of water and he would stick his head in and get the marble every time. Put a cracker six inches outside of his pen, and Bob would lay on his side, stick one paw through the wire, and get the cracker.

If I shot down two quail close together, he would retrieve both at one go. Bob would trail a covey of quail up to a fence, but instead of jumping the fence and scaring the quail, he would run down about seventy-five yards and go back and trail them. If he pointed a romp of quail and they started to run, he would go all the way around them. This would stop the birds, and they would be between Bob and me.

When I shot a covey late in the afternoon, they would scatter. But before nightfall they would do what we call "whistle" to get the covey together for the night. So if I shot at a covey late in the day, Bob would wait to hear one whistle and head for it, and when I got there, he would be standing on point. The next day he would head for it immediately. If I lost him on point, I'd just wait a few minutes. He would come back and start to whine, then lead me to the covey.

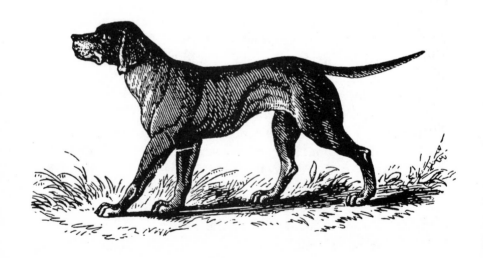

Buster Juggles Ducks

Submitted by Dr. R. G. MacKintosh, Yakima, Washington

Buster sat beside three of us in the duck blind. He shivered a little, and I did too. It was cold, yes, but part of the shiver was excitement. The northers were in! There was frost on the ground, skiff ice floated on the creek, and the tulles opposite the blind showed frost, though it was starting to melt just a little in the November sunrise. The wooden decoys swung quietly where he had put them. We crouched a bit and I made a clucking sound with my duck call and gave a long comeback call to a high and passing flock of mallards. Silence, then the whishing of wings.

We were ready. One bird fell dead into the icy water, but the other fell, spinning into the tulles on the far side and beyond the pond.

Buster plunged from the blind and into the skiff ice. He grabbed the dead duck and continued to the other side of the water, going right toward his mark. We could not see him, but from the thrashing sounds in the bulrushes we knew he was hot on the trail of the cripple.

Presently, Buster appeared, duck in his mouth, and went right to the edge of the water. He nosed the dead bird into the stream while still holding the cripple. Pushing it back to our side of Toppenish Creek, he left the bird lodged on the shore, brought in the wounded bird, then went back for the dead bird.

You know how dogs are—he never even bragged about his effort—but I surely did. I was glad to belong to a dog like that.

"All knowledge,
the totality of all questions
and all answers,
is contained in a dog."

—Franz Kafka, "Investigations of a Dog"

Courageous Dogs

Many dogs illustrate tremendous courage, vigilance, and faithfulness.

Shep's Amazing Vigil

Submitted by Dr. Robert P. Clark, Warsaw, Indiana

No one is sure when Shep's saga began, but it was probably in the late summer of 1936 in Montana. A shepherd had died, and as his remains were placed in the funeral car of the Great Northern Railroad, only one mourner was present at the depot, a sad-eyed collie with a broken heart.

The collie whined and scratched at the wooden gangway until the train carrying his master's casket pulled away and disappeared eastward-bound. Even then, Shep remained on the tracks for hours. He apparently believed that his master's departure was temporary. He dug a shelter under the depot and listened for the sound of incoming trains. Then he appeared on the platform, tail wagging, to survey disembarking passengers. He did this day after day, year after year.

Dogs at the depot had come and gone for years, so Shep's vigil went unnoticed at first. However, his constancy became apparent to the railroad men who fed him scraps and even made a place for him inside the depot. Comfort didn't change his vigil. Whatever the time or temperature, Shep was still the first to greet incoming trains daily. He sniffed at baggage and nosed the fingers of unloading travelers. He was often disappointed but never discouraged.

Soon Shep's story spread. A train conductor wrote the story down, the media picked it up, and by 1937 the collie had become a star. Great Northern passengers got off at the Fort Benton depot just to catch sight of the faithful dog. Many offered him a home, and people throughout the world sent gifts of money and food.

The money ultimately grew to a sizeable fortune and was eventually donated to the Montana School for the Deaf and Blind. Today, the "Shep Fund" provides everything from hearing aids to college tuition for children.

Shep kept his vigil at the depot for over five years. He met his last train on January 12, 1942. As usual, he waited between the tracks for its arrival. As it approached, Shep's stiff old legs couldn't move him off the tracks fast enough. Alas, Shep's vigil was over.

The trainmen buried Shep on a bluff over the depot, and built a concrete likeness of him as a tribute. For years, Great Northern illuminated the monument each night for the remarkably faithful dog.

A Million-Dollar Mutt

Submitted by H. E. Riggs, DVM, Mt. Gilead, Ohio

It was a warm spring day in rural Ohio. Marlow walked down the path to the barn, a trip he had taken many times through the years. He and his wife, Gertie, had fed and milked the cows, hayed the sheep, and completed their breakfast.

The old hay rack for the cows in the barnyard was falling apart, and Marlow had to fix it; he had put it off long enough. He had already placed some new boards under the rack last evening, and worked intently for a while. The cows, widely spaced in the area, looked with mild interest, but were mostly concerned with their mossing ration.

The project was shaping up. Suddenly, he was struck from behind by a great force that knocked him to the ground. The air was gone from his lungs. He lay there, helpless, dazed, and paralyzed. He could only glimpse the neighbor's red bull, horns sticking out like spikes on the side of his head, snorting, pawing, and now starting, with a twisted motion of the head, to finish him off.

Suddenly, he heard the shrill bark of a puppy. It was the one he had adopted from his neighbor as a favor, the mixed-breed little black one with splashes of white on his chest and paws. The puppy moved defiantly toward the enraged animal. What could a puppy do to help? The antagonized bull was in no mood to be irritated by such an unworthy foe. The bull swung around and charged at the noisy intruder, who wisely ran back under the barbed wire fence. Surely, thought Marlow, the little fellow would run away and hide.

Once more, the bull swung back to Marlow, who had managed a deep breath. But the yapping ball of fur returned, undaunted. The scene was repeated and again the puppy barely escaped.

Gertie's terrified scream prodded life into her husband. "Roll, Marlow, roll!" A third time the puppy made a swipe to torment and tease the bull, just as Marlow rolled under the fence. At last, the two were safe.

"Doc," Marlow told me, "He may be a mutt, but I wouldn't take a million dollars for him."

Dog of the Year

Submitted by Dr. Ronald Welby, Rapid City, Michigan

Late in the afternoon of April 3, 1956, a storm moved into our area with a strong wind and beating rain. Soon after the storm moved on, two small children were reported missing. The tiny village of Cedar Run was a heap of uprooted trees and homes, flattened buildings, smashed windows, and litter everywhere. A search ensued, and the children were ultimately found by their dog, Collie. The nine-year-old collie mix had searched for the pair, and was finally able to find them, pinned under the wreckage of their house. The dog then helped others drag them to safety.

For this display of intelligence and devotion, Collie received a trophy, a medal, two certificates of heroism, and was named Michigan's Dog of the Year.

A month after the tornado, Collie wasn't feeling well. After an examination, I discovered a two-and-a-half-inch piece of glass had punctured his skin and settled into Collie's abdomen. Collie had saved the children even while injured.

Following surgery, Collie made a full recovery, received another medal and certificate, and lived a long and normal life.

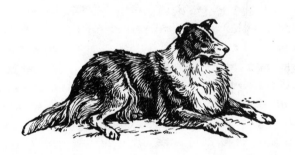

Perky and Jadxia

Submitted by Dr. V. R. Howie, Manson, Iowa

Amelia had grown up in a military family, living many different places around the world, but had always dreamed of being a farmer's wife. She loved animals. Now she was living in western Nebraska with her new husband, Kerry. It was like a dream come true. It was also here, on Grandpa League's ranch, that she learned not only just how much she loved animals, but that they also return love, sometimes in unexpected ways.

Kerry had taken the tractor and gone to the field to get a load of dirt to build flower beds, so Amelia busied herself with the dishes and cleaning the kitchen. As she scurried around, she paused to listen. Grandpa League's dog, Perky, was outside the window crying. That's strange, Amelia thought, Perky doesn't usually cry without a reason. But she continued to clean the kitchen. A few minutes later, she heard Perky crying again, so she decided that she should see what was wrong. When she got to the yard, she could hear Kerry's tractor running. She looked in that direction and saw that the tractor was upside down. Terror-stricken, she rushed to the tractor to find Kerry pinned under the overturned tractor, his legs trapped under a wheel. The tractor was still running and it was still in gear. Despite her frantic efforts, she could not shut off the tractor. The wheel that was in the air continued to spin. Amelia called 911. "Where are you?" the operator asked. Amelia responded, "You will have to find me. I am on the Howard League ranch." Then she rushed back to Kerry's side. The rescue crew arrived and, after forty-five minutes, Kerry was on his way to the hospital emergency room. A miracle: Kerry turned out to be fine. Not a single bone had been broken, but he would be sore for a few days. No less miraculous was the fact that Perky had alerted Amelia that something was wrong when the tractor fell on Kerry, crying for her not only once but twice, until she responded.

Jadxia was just a puppy when Amelia bought her while performing at the Ohio Renaissance Festival. The puppy had been named for the Star Trek character, Jadxia Dax. She was half German shepherd and half husky, but you might have thought she was also half pack rat. Since she'd come to

Nebraska, she would bring everything imaginable to Amelia—ice chunks from the cattle's watering troughs, dried cow patties, and corn stalks, among other things. If Amelia wasn't available, Jadxia would put her findings in her doghouse. One time, Amelia unloaded groceries from the car and found only one can of orange juice in the bag, whereas she'd been charged for two. The next day, she found the undamaged can of juice in Jadxia's house. Then there was the time Amelia heard a terrible racket outside, and went out to discover Jadxia trying to get a deer—head, antlers, and all—into her house, perhaps as a wall decoration to put above the fireplace in her den?

Amelia's brother, Dan, had driven out from Minnesota to spend one Thanksgiving weekend, and they had had a wonderful day of horseback riding. As they charged down the steep embankment and headed for home at the end of the day, Dan's glasses suddenly flew from his face. Kerry, Amelia, and Dan all dismounted to find the glasses. Hand in hand, they traversed up and down the hill, searching for nearly an hour but to no avail. It was getting cold and dark, so they decided that if they didn't find the glasses on the next pass, they would just have to forget them. But Dan really needed them to see for his drive back to Minnesota. In frustration, Amelia turned to

Jadxia and chastised, "You always bring me all this useless junk, why don't you bring me Dan's glasses?" Failing to find the glasses, they returned to the horses for the ride home. As they were preparing to mount up, Amelia called for Jadxia, who came bounding through the tall grass with Dan's glasses held gently in her mouth.

Needless to say, Perky and Jadxia hold very special places in the hearts of all the members of Kerry and Amelia's families.

Two men were sitting on a bench. One man saw a dog by the other and asked if his dog bit. The man said no. So the other man reached down to pet the dog and the dog bit him. "I thought you said your dog doesn't bite."

"That's not my dog."

Smart Dogs

Some dogs are smarter than we realize; just smart enough to have other dogs, or even people, do jobs for them.

Sparky, an Ice Dog

Submitted by Dr. Blais and Roy Baukol, Indiana, Pennsylvania

We received a Labrador pup and called her Sparky. (We wanted to call her Spark Plug because she can get from 0 to 60 in 2.2 seconds.) She loves ice cubes. When she was with us about two months, she discovered that my wife takes a glass of ice cubes to bed, and at the same time she found out that we have touch lamps on the night stands that can be pressed from one to three times for brightness. Every night it's the same routine:

the dog comes into the bedroom, presses the lamp with her nose three times, sits down, and waits for her ice cube. She does this three times, then my wife says "no more," and she lies down for the night.

Sam Could Tell Time

Submitted by Dr. Robert C. Glover, New Port Richey, Florida

Our dog, Sam, lived until he was 15 years of age—a real senior canine citizen. Sam was very smart and very opinionated; also he could tell time very well. When I retired, Sam was one year of age. Enjoying retirement meant for me a happy hour at 5 p.m., just in time for the 5:00 news. Usually some peanuts or popcorn went along with the libations. Every day at 4:45 p.m., Sam stood by my big red chair in which I enjoyed my five o'clock happy hour. If I didn't show up, he would bark until I assumed my evening ritual. Sam knew he would get a treat at that time.

Sam enjoyed sitting alone in a float chair in our swimming pool. He would bark near the pool until someone placed the float chair in the pool. Sam would swim to the chair, crawl in and spend hours snoozing and keeping cool. He didn't want anyone in the chair with him. What a life!

A Slam Dunk for Toby

Submitted by Dr. Candy Lewis, Lakeside, California

Toby and Winston, two springer spaniels, live with my mother. Toby, generally considered to be the smarter of the two, loves nylabones (chew bones made of nylon). Winston, a tennis ball freak, especially likes to dunk the balls in the toilet or a puddle of water before having a long, satisfying chew. One night, for unknown reasons, Winston decided to try the Nylabone, much to Toby's dismay. Finding no way to get the Nylabone from Winston, Toby left the room, went to the kitchen, and picked up a tennis ball. He took the ball to the water dish and dropped it in. After a moment, he retrieved the ball and went back into the family room, lying down near Winston. For a few minutes, he chewed loudly on the soaked tennis ball and then "lost interest." He got up and nonchalantly walked around Winston. Winston, thinking he was seizing the moment, got up and lunged for the deserted tennis ball. Toby grabbed his beloved Nylabone and ran off to a corner to chew it contentedly. The very deliberate dunking of the ball into the water dish is what makes this story so unique—Toby never placed his toys in the water, before or since.

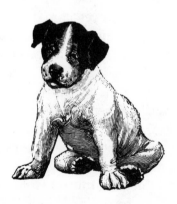

Susie

Submitted by Dr. William G. Gross, Jacksonville, Illinois

One evening, I went to visit with Susie, a twelve-year-old golden Labrador, and her owner, Jim Vierae, after caring for some farm animals in the barn. Jim and I were seated in the dining area near a refrigerator. The refrigerator had a towel tied to the door handle. Susie was lying on the floor with her head between her legs, eyes closed, apparently napping. Jim and I were in a conversation and he asked if I would like a soda or beer. I replied that a beer sounded good, as this was my last call of the day. Jim said, "Susie, Doc would like a beer." Immediately, Susie jumped up, walked to the refrigerator, pulled on the towel to open the door, reached in, and grasped a can of beer in her mouth. She walked directly to me to deliver the beer. Then she walked back to Jim's chair, laid down, and resumed the same position as before.

He told her, "Susie, I think I would like a soda," and she repeated the same procedure as before, only with a soda.

Susie's telephone routine was a similar procedure. When

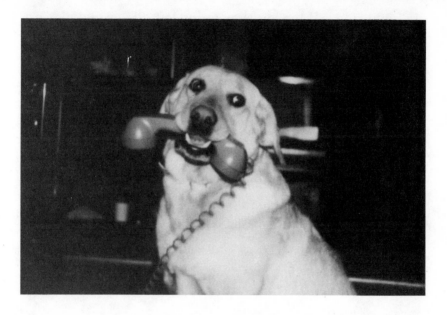

the phone rang, Jim would say, "Susie, bring me the headset," which she did. After Jim completed his call, he would say, "Susie, take the headset back," which she would do promptly. Even when Susie could hear the phone ring, she wouldn't respond unless Jim told her to do so. She could tell the difference between shoes. Jim always placed the right shoe on the right side and the left shoe to the left. She would pick up the right or left, as directed.

Jim had five dogs to feed. Jim once called, "It's feeding time. Go fetch the bucket." His yard had five one-gallon ice cream pails with wire hole handles scattered about. Susie would pick up one, then another, then a third bucket in her mouth. When trying to add a fourth, she would drop one of the buckets. Jim remarked, "Susie, remember you have to stack them." To my amazement, Susie looked up at Jim and then started putting one bucket after another on top of each other, until all the buckets were in the stack. She then brought them to Jim to be filled with dog food.

Bilingual Bob

Submitted by Dr. Stanton E. Bower, San Luis Obispo, California

Bob belonged to Mr. and Mrs. Dick Kelsey of See Canyon, an area in San Luis Obispo County. Bob understood English, and all of us who knew him knew he understood what we were saying. He even understood whether we were talking to him or not. Mr. Kelsey was a farmer with an apple orchard. On some days he would have to drive to town in the morning instead of working around the farm and orchard. Bob always laid against the wall just inches from the kitchen door. Mr. and Mrs. Kelsey ate breakfast in the kitchen. On the mornings when Dick was going out to work, Bob would beat him out the door and run all over the place ahead of him. However, on the mornings when Dick was going into town, Bob would not move from where he was lying. He simply listened to the conversation at the breakfast table and knew what Dick was going to do. On Bob's final visit to the hospital, due to a foxtail penetrating his abdominal cavity, we did not have to lead or handle him in the hospital; we simply told him what to do. We'd open the cage door and tell him to go into the treatment room or the surgery, or to wait in the hall or the ward, and he always did exactly what we asked.

Extraordinary Escapes

Somehow, some way, even the most obedient dogs can escape from leashes, fences, and locked doors.

The Cold, Cruel World

Submitted by Dr. W. P. Berner, San Rafael, California

At one point during construction to remodel our animal hospital, our animal security was totally compromised, and if a dog got out of his exercise run or was loose for any reason, it had the opportunity to escape our facility. Although I warned our staff about our vulnerability a dog escaped, running full speed down the street.

Later that day, a client came in and said there was a dog out in front acting funny. When we went out to check, there was our lost, wild dog, just waiting for someone to open the door so he could get back inside. I suppose the outside world was not as exciting as it seemed.

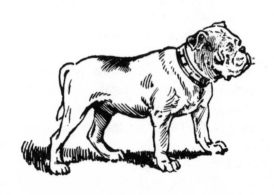

The End of a Friendship

Submitted by Dr. W. P. Berner, San Rafael, California

Mr. Wurzburg, a fellow country-club golfer, owned a large, mixed-breed dog by the name of Duke. His children were grown, so he and his wife traveled a lot, occasionally bringing Duke in to board at our hospital. The Wurzburgs lived across town with many obstacles between their residence and our hospital, including the entrance to Highway 101. When the couple went on a trip and left Duke with neighbors who fed and took care of him instead of boarding him with us, he would run away and travel across the various obstacles ending up at the hospital. Naturally, we took him in and called the owners when they returned. After about the sixth time or so that this occurred, the Wurzburgs got tired of retrieving Duke and suggested we chase him off when he appeared. I can still see Duke running across the street, hiding behind the wheel of a car and waiting and watching us to see if he wasn't welcomed back. He tried sneaking back in a few times, but each time we had to shoo him away, as ordered.

That was the last we saw of Duke. He was a very entertaining dog. We truly had lost a friend, and I'm sure he felt the same way.

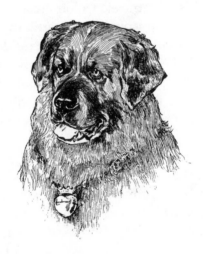

Family Dogs

Some dogs have natural nurturing qualities, whether it's for other puppies, other species, or people. Here are some of the more charming stories I received.

Napping, Not Yapping
Submitted by Clifford T. Kumamoto, Honolulu, Hawaii

Momi, my Chihuahua, was born with a lot of natural intelligence. When she was a puppy, I taught her the basic obedience commands. However, there were two she taught herself.

The first was her way of notifying me that the phone or doorbell was ringing. She would bark until I answered the call. Even if I was taking a shower, she would run into the bathroom and start barking until I acknowledged her action.

The more interesting trait she demonstrated was more of maternal instinct, although she never had a litter of pups herself. Most of us think of Chihuahuas as a snappy and yappy breed, but when a baby was laid down for a nap, Momi would

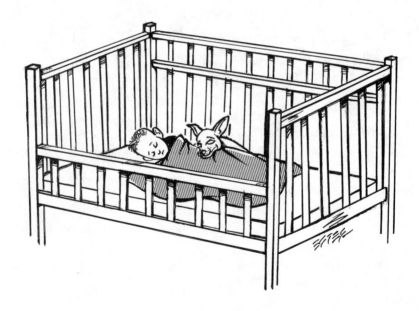

jump onto the bed or sofa and lie right up against the baby's body to give it warmth. She would not allow anyone to come near the infant, and would growl and curl her lips if any person tried. However, when the baby woke up and started crying, she would jump down and let us know that it was okay to attend to the baby.

August the Aussie

Submitted by Dr. Candy Lewis, Lakeside, California

My Australian shepherd, August, was a C-section pup. I raised him with a lot of handling as I started my second year of vet school. He had almost no sight in his left eye from birth, but that never held him down. He was talked to from the time he was born, and knew as many words as many five-year-old children.

One of August's favorite things was to help me raise orphan kittens, and as soon as they were old enough to move around, he would bring them back when they moved too far.

His most memorable ability was the way he knew the names of all of my other animals. He could find any of them, including the hamster who escaped from his cage the first night we had him. I asked August where the hamster was and he went looking until he found him hiding in the back of a closet under an old sheet. He would routinely find the cats and rabbits when asked. When we moved to Lakeside and acquired Mach, a desert tortoise, August would look for him in our one-acre plot.

Poochie the Protector

Submitted by Dr. Bob Stine, Pensacola, Florida

One Sunday I decided to bring an ill calf home with me in order to more easily feed it and to provide a more comfortable environment for both of us. The patient was responding favorably to my treatment but was still unable to walk. As I positioned the calf in a shady area in the backyard, my female boxer named Poochie appeared and proceeded to check things out. While the sniffing process was going on, I gave her instructions to look out for the calf. After lunch, I looked out the window and was surprised to see a neighborhood dog approaching the calf. Immediately, I headed for the door to supervise things, but Poochie came bolting out from her station under the house, bowled the intruder over with her shoulder, placed her front foot on her subject, and, after the proper submissive response was obtained, allowed him to get up and slink off. The vigil continued on into the afternoon. Poochie allowed her Chihuahua playmate from next door to explore the calf with close supervision.

No new threats to her charge occurred until my three boys, ages two to five years, awoke from their naps and approached my patient. Poochie was now facing a dilemma. She loved the boys and was their protector, but she didn't really trust them with the calf. I watched her from a window as she placed herself between the children and the calf, and gently nudged them away while looking at the house in search of reinforcement. Her look of relief was very apparent when I came outside and gave her help with the kids.

Poochie had demonstrated great capability in understanding her assignment and judgment in handling difficult problems. She recognized the need to protect the calf, allowed her trusted friend to approach it, dealt harshly with a dog that she considered a threat, and exercised good responsibility when the boys approached her charge.

Dogs Keep Dad out of Doghouse

Submitted by Dr. Dale Kaplan-Stein, Gainesville, Florida

When my daughters were sixteen months and three years old respectively, we had eight dogs. None of them were trained for anything special but were merely well-loved pets. We lived on eight acres, and our neighbors had just as much land.

One day I got sick and was running a fever of about 104, so my husband had to watch the kids. Later that day, I awoke and went to check on them. To my horror, I found my husband asleep, the three-year-old watching television, and the baby gone. I checked our pool, but thank God we had a pool fence, so she wasn't there. She had wandered down our driveway and into our neighbor's yard, about five hundred yards away. There she was, sitting and "reading" their newspaper, with all eight of our dogs in a circle around her. I have no doubt that they were guarding her and knew exactly what they were doing. My only mistake was not taking a picture.

Wally and the Wall Key

Submitted by Adrian Broderick, age ten (granddaughter of Dr. Jules Silder)

Wally, my red, male Australian shepherd, is *extremely* smart and very pretty. My brother, Jordan, is an early riser. Usually he is the first one up on weekends. Wally always has to go to the bathroom, first thing in the morning. One morning, Jordan had to tend to his bathroom needs first. We have a key that is on a plastic Oreo cookie key chain that we use to open the door. Wally knows that this is the key to use to go out, and it hangs on a hook about one and a half feet above the floor— easy to get for a big dog like Wally.

So, while Jordan was in the bathroom, Wally got the "cookie" key off the wall and went to the bathroom door, which was open a crack. He stuck his nose in the crack, went in, and put the key on Jordan's lap while he was sitting on the toilet. I don't think Jordan was too crazy about Wally's visit, but this way Wally's needs could be attended to as well.

Brownie, Herder and Hunter

Submitted by Vyrle D. Stauffer, DVM, Arvada, Colorado

Brownie was of mixed ancestry, mostly shepherd, and was, of course, a dirty-brown color. He was a home-trained sheep herder of unusual ability, and was a champion in the eyes of my family, although he had never won a trophy.

My family raised the sheep on the ranges of Idaho. Sheep dogs were an indispensable part of these operations. A group of three or four dogs accompanied each herd of 2,000 or more. Brownie was the leader of the pack, and had taught numerous other young dogs the secret of herding sheep. As soon as school was out in the spring, we would accompany the sheep out on the range land about fifty miles from the home ranch. We would remain there until school started again in the fall. Each morning, the sheep were turned from the bed-ground to the area they were to graze, and in the late afternoon were turned back to the camp. When an area had been sufficiently grazed, the camp was moved to a new field area about three miles away.

All this maneuvering required the assistance of the dogs, directed by my father. Signals were given to them, by whistles and hand signals, as to what they were supposed to do. Frequently, the tall sagebrush would obstruct the view of the dog from the herder. In such circumstances, Brownie would jump in the air, above the brush to receive the hand signals, which he carried out quickly. In camp one day, we found an owl's nest that had two chicks in it. They were obviously abandoned, so we decided to feed them. What do they eat? Well, wild rodents, of course; in that area, ground squirrel was most available. Brownie turned out to be the best provider of rodents. As the owls matured and began to vocalize, one came up with the word "meat" as clearly as a person would pronounce it. Whenever he would shout out meat, Brownie would start hunting for squirrels and lay them near the owl's perch.

Shep Worked Until the Cows Came Home

Submitted by D. Norman Ganlick, Charleston, South Carolina

While I was studying veterinary medicine, I had the opportunity to work on a small dairy farm near the town of Eatonville, Washington. The owner had done his own dog training, and Shep, an Australian shepherd dog, was a natural, with highly developed herding instincts.

At this dairy farm, cattle-driving by people on foot was a waste of time, and the cattle could not be relied on to come in for their milking.

Every morning and evening at milking time, Shep would wait at the milk house door, his eyes filled with obvious excitement, and his body tense with anticipation. At the words "Go and get them," spoken by any of the three farmhands, Shep would race out into the pasture, and within twenty to thirty minutes, he had the cows entering the lane leading to the barn. Shep would slip under the fence and race to the end of the lane, where he would watch while the cows came in through the gate. If all the cows came through, Shep would expect some well-deserved praise. However, if one or more of the cows were missing at the gate, Shep would race back into the pasture, and in a short time he would retrieve the missing cows. He never had to go back more than once, and he always knew when every cow had been accounted for. He also knew which of the cows were most likely to hide out. Shep lived for his work and loved it. I only wished that he could have learned to milk those cows and spare me the task!

A Furry Baseball Fan

Submitted by John M. Gamberdella, Branford, Connecticut

When a client mentioned that his old Labrador, Augie, enjoyed TV and actually watched the tube with him, I said "You're kidding!"

"No, I'm not kidding," he replied. "In fact, when we watch a baseball game together and the batter gets a hit, he actually runs behind the TV set looking for the ball."

What's a Dalmation's
favorite type of dance?

The Polka.

Hightailing to the Hospital

Sometimes we wonder if dogs really need us at all. After all, they can even go to the doctor's by themselves. Here are a few stories of very smart—and independent—dogs.

Sandy, Our Lovable Nuisance

Submitted by Don Krushak, DVM, MPH, San Francisco, California

Sandy was a crossbred (mostly German shepherd) male dog with an engaging personality. When he was happy, his tongue dangled from the side of his laughing mouth, and he would slobber on anyone who paid attention to his antics. His owners traveled a lot, so Sandy was a frequent boarder at our hospital. In fact, we soon became his second home, although he preferred to think of it as his primary one.

If his owners let him out of the house, he would make a beeline for our hospital and greet all comers. In time, he learned how to depress the thumb latch of the waiting room door, then cavort around the room, making all welcome. We soon learned to recognize the sound of his nails on the tile floor, and upon opening the inner door, he greeted the attendants with a leap and kiss as he sped for the kennel, his home away from home.

His favorite companion was the kennel cat, Suzy. With a quick bark, Sandy would select an empty cage and was soon joined by Suzy—they were inseparable. We never learned whether he came to see Suzy or us.

So that he couldn't enter the waiting room when no one else was around, we changed the latch to a door knob. However, he would lay at the door and wait for the first client to open it. The steady customers soon learned he was harmless, and just happy to be there to see them. New clients would tell us about the dog guarding the doorway so they couldn't enter. We assured them: just pat him, shove him aside, and quickly get inside. And don't let him in!

Eventually, we had to report to his master that Sandy was

becoming a nuisance. He attempted to break Sandy's habitual runaways by chaining him in the yard. However, when Sandy was in the house and one of the children entered or left, he saw his opportunity and was off to visit his pal, Suzy, and his favorite veterinary hospital friends.

The Tale of Fox Tail

Submitted by Victor H. Austin, DVM, MS, Westlake Village,
California

One day, a beautiful, healthy-looking male golden retriever
appeared at the closed glass front door of the veterinary
hospital in Ventura, California. The doctor I was working for
was not in the office at that time, and I questioned the
receptionist as to what the dog was doing. She hadn't noticed
him until I asked the question, but she immediately replied,
"Open the door and let Fred in."

Fred walked in when I opened the door, walked to the
nearest vacant exam room, placed his front paws on the exam
table, and waited to be lifted up, which the attendant did. Fred
positioned himself on the table (head end towards the hanging
otoscope) and tilted his head to the side. Joe said, "Look in his
ear." He steadied Fred's head while I looked in and saw a large,
fresh foxtail awn, something common with many open lots
and no leash laws. I immediately removed it.

Fred jumped to the floor, went to the front door, and waited
for Joe to open it. He looked like he was smiling as he trotted

out the door and down the street toward home. Jennie, the receptionist, picked up the phone and called the dog's owner, Mrs. Taylor. "Fred was just here—the foxtail was in his right ear. Watch for any trouble." Mrs. Taylor thanked her and said, "Bill us, as usual."

Another story not related to intelligence, just a funny one. My partner sent a dog home after an office call and inadvertently didn't take out the rectal thermometer. The upset owner called to complain, "You know you left a thermometer in my dog?" Quickly thinking, my partner said "Oh, I meant to call you. I wanted to know what his temperature was at home. Will you read it for me please?" She did!

Leo Takes a Trip to the Hospital All by Himself

Used by permission of the *Garden Grove Journal*

Leo Buckalew went for a walk Monday, fell in with a rough bunch, got in a fight, got chewed up pretty bad, and took himself to the hospital.

Sound remarkable? Well, this Leo is a three-and-a-half-year-old basset hound, and his trip to the vet has his owner and the doctor still shaking their heads.

"I've been practicing veterinary medicine for twenty-eight years, and I've never seen anything like it," said Dr. Les Malo of Garden Grove Boulevard.

"I told my daughter," said Leo's owner, Charles Buckalew, Jr., "and she doesn't believe me."

Apparently, Charles and Leo were going for a walk from their home on Pleasant Street when Leo tangled with another dog who Charles described as a pit bull. The other dog was driven off, but Leo, somewhat worse for the wear with many cuts and bites, took off.

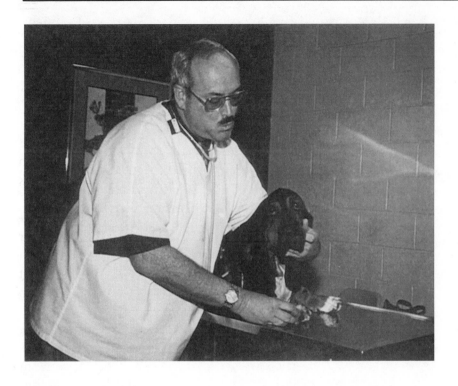

But where to?

Over at the Garden Grove Dog and Cat Hospital, two veterinary technicians were taking a break in the parking lot when they watched this low-slung dog walk up, visit a bush, and then present himself at the entrance.

Seeing the dog's wounds, the employees of the pet hospital let him inside, where he walked through the reception room, down the hall into surgery, and sat waiting to be treated. After a while, up walked Charles, asking "Have you seen my dog?"

Leo had been a patient at the hospital before, and he evidently remembered both the mission and the geography of the vet's office. "He knew right where to go," marveled Dr. Malo. "He's a very intelligent dog," said Buckalew.

So much so, perhaps, that next time maybe Leo will drive.

Judge Goes Hunting, Then Hunts for a Vet

Submitted by Dr. R. G. MacKintosh, Yakima, Washington

One afternoon, as clients came to the clinic bringing their patients in for treatment, a springer spaniel insisted on coming in from the street. No owner appeared with him who seemed responsible for this animal. We were located downtown and quite a ways from the residential area of our town. Dogs don't usually like being treated, so I put him outside the door and had to repeat the process three or four times. He just insisted on coming in.

My father—the good doctor—looked at the weed-matted and bedraggled old character and said, "Bring him in and clean up those mats and cockle burrs." He was a mess. As I was clipping off the mats and burrs from the dog's ears, he flinched. My father, in the meantime, called an old friend of his on the phone. Billy Treneer, the local blacksmith, had lost his dog, again, and we had found him.

It seems that this spaniel, "Judge" by name, had a hunting

companion and friend, Hunky Shaw's setter. Periodically, both dogs would go off for a hunt. To do this, Judge had to go almost a mile, past eight blocks of houses—and a lot of other dogs—to find the Shaw dog and talk him into a hunt. Then the two went about three miles south down a busy street to get to a favorite area south of the Ahtanum Creek, where they had a good chance of finding game. These two old partners had done this before. They were just good old boys like their owners.

The other times they had hunted, returned home, and hadn't needed help. This time the setter went home, but Judge had remembered where he had been helped before, so he went in a different direction, some three and a half miles northeast, and crossed the railroad switching yard. He went twenty-five streets east of his normal haunts to get the foxtails removed from his ear canals and to get the cockle burrs from his coat.

My father asked Mr. Treneer if he wanted to pick up Judge after work at the smithy. Billy just said, "If he's fixed up, just turn him out the door. He'll come home. I'll send you a check."

Hightailing a Foxtail to the Hospital

Submitted by Roy I. Hostetler, DVM, Seattle, Washington

While in veterinary practice in Goldendale, Washington, I met up with a cute little black cocker spaniel who had the misfortune of living in a foxtail area. As a result, she made numerous trips to my office, in spite of clipping her coat short.

Most dogs under similar circumstances have to be carried, or dragged, to the operating table. But this dog, after a couple of trips with foxtails lodged in her ears, would go to her owner's car, tip her head sideways toward the problem ear, and whine for attention. When the car door was opened, she would immediately jump into the car.

Upon arriving at the hospital, the dog would go straight to the examining room and look up to be placed on the operating table. Most dogs have to be forcibly put on the table and possibly anesthetized before a successful operation can be accomplished. This little dog would sit perfectly still and whine, but not move, while the offending beards were removed. Upon completion of the operation, she would turn, put her front paws against me, and lick me on the face.

Biff Keeps His Appointment

Submitted by Norman L. Garlick, DVM, Charleston, South Carolina

Biff was a large dog of dubious ancestry, who had the run of a suburban section of Tacoma, Washington, where I was in practice. Biff had the misfortune of accumulating grass seed awns in the hair between his toes. His owners brought him in with a severely lame left front leg, which was considerably swollen. I removed the awn, irrigated the tract, applied suitable medication, and bandaged the foot. Old Biff took it well, and I discharged the patient with the request that he be brought back the following Tuesday for a change of dressing and further treatment, if necessary.

The following Tuesday, as I arrived at the hospital in the morning, I noted a dog up on his hind feet looking into the window of the front door of the hospital. I recognized the bandage and the dog, opened the door, and he came in with me. I placed him in a kennel, pending treatment. There was no sign of his owner. He obligingly sat on the examination table without restraint while I changed the dressing and rebandaged the foot. We expected his owners to come in and claim him. By mid-afternoon the owners had not called for him. We placed a telephone call to them with the news that Biff was ready to be picked up. The owner exclaimed with considerable amazement that they had been looking for Biff all day, knowing he was to be returned for follow-up treatment, but were not able to find him. I related the fact that Biff was at the door at opening hour, and was eager to enter with me as I opened for the day. Biff had traveled more than three miles on his own the day he was to return for care!

Big Red's Lame Excuse

Submitted by Seymour Glasofer, DVM, Newport News, Virginia

A middle-aged couple owned a handsome Chesapeake Bay retriever named "Big Red." Both owners worked, and were usually not with the dog during the day.

Big Red was brought to my office one day with a minor leg lesion, causing a slight foreleg limp. The lesion was treated and a bandage applied. Then the patient received much attention and petting from the owners, with many expressions such as "Poor, poor Red has a bad foot."

The dog made a very uneventful recovery from this condition, but it wasn't long before he began appearing frequently for treatment. No pathology was ever found that could account for the lameness of any of these visits; however, on one trip to the office a skin infection on one leg needed bandaging. How he loved that! Big Red showed so much pleasure and tail-wagging over this minor medical treatment that even his owners suspected a plot.

From that day on, at least once each week, Big Red came by

himself (a distance of about one mile) to the clinic, appearing with one foreleg elevated. When Red arrived, we put a bandage on a limb (it made absolutely no difference which limb) and our patient would dash home to receive a "poor dog has a bad foot"—plus some treat to help ease his "pain."

There was no doubt Big Red was a hypochondriac. He was such an appealing one that we were willing to play along with his imagined injuries for a while. But finally we were afraid Big Red might cry wolf once too often. We were also worried about his traveling to the clinic unattended and being exposed to traffic; he might arrive actually lame and no one would believe him.

For his own sake, we had to stop bandaging our attention seeker. We advised his owners to give Big Red lots of love and a little less sympathy, and most of all, to direct their attention to matters other than his "lameness."

Sally—Our Adopted Dog

Submitted by Dr. J. R. Saunders, San Antonio, Texas

A small brown and tan, long-haired dog, a very emaciated and obviously post-lactational female, once appeared at our clinic. We were on a highway at the edge of town, a convenient place for people to unload unwanted pets, and so were not surprised.

Mr. Winslow, my helper, a retired, kindly gentleman, fed and watered our guest. The next day the dog was still around, and he suggested that we take her into the clinic and clean her up a little. He clipped out her mats of long hair and gave her a bath. We also obtained a fecal specimen, checked her for parasites, and started her on vaccinations. After about ten days, I took her home to my family. She had been named Sally by then.

About a year later, our wonderful pet Sally did not come for her morning food. We called and looked all around our immediate neighborhood, but no Sally.

When I reached my office that morning, Mr. Winslow said

that Sally was waiting at the door of the clinic when he arrived. I reclaimed her and took her home when I went for lunch.

The next morning, Sally was missing again. Since Mr. Winslow usually arrived about a half-hour earlier than I, I telephoned the office and, sure enough, she was there again, waiting. He also told me that she felt hot and had a swelling above one eye. After examining her, I determined that she had a fractured and abscessed upper-third premolar.

After the tooth was extracted and the abscess drained, we kept her in the clinic a few days until her appetite returned.

We had Sally for several years after that, and she only left home when she went with the family, and was a wonderful loving pet.

Lessons to Learn from Dogs

1. Never pass up the opportunity for a joy ride.

2. Eat with gusto and enthusiasm.

3. Avoid biting when a simple growl will do.

A Nose for Direction

As any dog owner can tell you, dogs have a magnificent sense of direction. Following are a few stories about dogs with an incredible kind of connection to their masters; those dogs will find home against any obstacle.

A Dog's Devotion

Submitted by Norman Garlick, DVM, Charleston, South Carolina

I was in general veterinary practice at Tacoma, Washington, where there was much ship-building activity, and workers were coming in from all over the United States to work in the shipyards. One day, a man came into the hospital reception room carrying a gaunt, medium-sized black dog of mixed spaniel breed. The man had tears in his eyes, and the dog was obviously exhausted. Its paws were a bloody mess, the pads being totally worn off. As the patient was admitted, we began to get the story.

The man and his family had just traveled from Kansas to Tacoma to work in the shipyards. He had reluctantly decided that he would have to leave his dog in Kansas, and had placed him with another family there.

The day he brought the dog to us he had just left work. It was less than a week since he had arrived in Tacoma. As he walked out the gate toward his car, he was met by his dog who he had left in Kansas! He was totally overwhelmed with emotion. He gathered him up in his arms and brought him straight to us to provide the care he would need to recover. There was every reason to believe the man's account—the condition of the dog was consistent with a journey of almost 2,000 miles on foot, most of the way without adequate water, and probably little or no food. The dog made an excellent recovery and was soon restored to his master, this time for life.

From Surf to Home Turf

Submitted by Dr. Keith Richter, Rancho Santa Fe, California

When Duke, a wonderful German shorthaired pointer, was first adopted from the humane society by his new owner, Steve, he was taken to his new home in Santa Monica. Two hours later, Steve drove Duke to the Santa Monica beach, approximately five miles from home. After playing for a few hours on the beach, Duke and Steve got separated. Steve looked frantically for a few hours for his new friend, but eventually gave up. Dejectedly he drove home. There, waiting for him at his front door was Duke. He somehow found his way home—over five miles to a home he had only been in once for a couple of hours. Duke and Steve have been best friends since then, for almost seventeen years. Not only is he a great dog, a wonderful patient, but he is also the oldest German short-haired pointer I have ever seen (over 17½ years)!

Kuhfus "Nose" the Way

Submitted by Dr. J. R. Saunders, San Antonio, Texas

Kuhfus was an Irish setter—intelligent, friendly, and a good hunting dog. He enjoyed going to the farm with the boys. Sometimes, he would hunt along the way; the other times, he would choose to ride in the wagon.

One time during the cotton-picking season we had a group of seven or eight boys who wanted to get an early start in order to put in a good day's work. No hunting on this day, so we decided to leave Kuhfus at home.

We were going to leave home before daylight, drive the five miles to the farm, and cook breakfast after we got there. We prepared a grub box consisting of bacon, eggs, bread, jelly, butter, etc. We hitched the horses to the wagon, loaded the grub along with the boys, tied old Kuhfus to a tree, and gave instructions to the folks to turn him loose after we'd been gone awhile. All this time, Kuhfus had been with us and apparently listening to our plans. He had a mind of his own. What did we find at the farm but Kuhfus sitting beside the fireplace with a stick of wood in his mouth. He had traveled the five miles by detour without being seen by our group, and no doubt thought that if he beat us there and gathered wood for the fire, he could stay with the boys without a scolding. He got no scolding but a generous portion of bacon, eggs, bread, butter, and jelly for breakfast.

Memorable Tales

Rex and Ole Dan
Submitted by Nicholas H. Booth, DVM, Ph.D.

I grew up on a dairy farm in the 1930s near Hannibal, Missouri, not far from the Mississippi River. All through elementary and high school, I arose at 4:00 every morning to deliver milk in glass bottles to the front door of the homes in Hannibal. Everyone expected to have their milk delivered by 6 A.M.

At one house, not too far from Mark Twain's home, a black and white dog named Dan barked at my heels and chased me every morning, as I ran the milk to the front porch. My father disliked all of the barking dogs we encountered each morning, particularly those that tried to bite me, as well as the front tire of our delivery truck.

On every Fourth of July, my dad looked forward to throwing cherry-bomb firecrackers from the truck window at dogs that ran for the front wheel of the truck. The explosion of the "bomb" proved to be the best deterrent for dogs that chased vehicles.

When my father went to the door every month to collect money for the delivered milk, he often informed the customers about their unruly pets. Although many of the customers would keep their dogs inside or tethered, there were some that continued to let their dogs run free. This was the case with Ole Dan.

My father kept telling Dan's master that something needed to be done, or he would discontinue deliveries. There had been other complaints about Ole Dan, and his master didn't know what to do with him. He said he didn't want to shoot him, and had the idea that we might take him to our dairy farm as a watchdog. We already had a fox terrier named Rex, who was just bought from my grandfather, but after a family discussion, we decided Rex needed a canine companion. Rex did not appear to be too happy after leaving my grandfather's place. Perhaps another dog like Ole Dan would lift his spirits.

Consequently, we acquired Ole Dan for Rex. However, I believe my dad actually obtained Ole Dan to prevent him from being shot. My father gave the impression of being tough and rugged, but beneath it all he was a good-hearted person.

When Rex was first introduced to Ole Dan, he curled his upper lip and snarled. My Dad decided that it was necessary to confine Ole Dan in the woodshed until Rex was ready to give him a better reception. After about a week of confinement, with short visits, Rex didn't curl his lip and snarl as much. Ole Dan always appeared to be exuberant when he saw Rex. Within two weeks, you could never have guessed that Rex ever had a dislike for Ole Dan.

After Rex's complete acceptance of Ole Dan, he took him out into the fields to hunt for rabbits. Ole Dan, being a city dog, had never hunted animals. One day, on a rabbit-hunting trip, I saw Rex and Ole Dan chasing one full speed toward a brush pile. The rabbit went into the pile with both dogs close behind. Rex circled the brush pile to see if the rabbit would run out the other side. To my amazement, Ole Dan jumped on top of the pile and began leaping up and down to make the rabbit run out. Sure enough, after a few moments, the rabbit ran out and toward another brush pile. Rex and Ole Dan were off in pursuit. It seemed that the rabbit enjoyed the chase as much as the dogs.

An Unexpected Lesson

Reprinted with permission from *The Prairie Practitioner*

The first holiday I was ever on duty was July 4, 1964. My first call came at 6:00 A.M. A couple from out of town were on their way to the clinic with a dog that had been run over. We had company, so I asked my father-in-law, and a young boy who was working for my in-laws, if they wanted to come along. They did, so when we pulled up to the clinic, the couple was already there. I gave the keys to my father-in-law to open up as I went to get the dog.

As I walked to the car, I immediately noticed that the young lady who was holding the dog didn't have any clothes on. Instead of embarrassing her, I told her I would meet her boyfriend in the office. However, she walked right in and set the dog on the examining table. She reluctantly let go, and backed away. In the meantime, her boyfriend brought her clothes and she proceeded to dress while I examined the dog. As she started to dress, the young boy walked in the office. I'll never forget his face; he learned a lesson other than veterinary care.

A Love Story

Submitted by Wallace Adrian, DVM, Hermosa, South Dakota

King, a German shepherd, had been mistaken for a stray, and had been shot through the back leg, completely severing his Achilles tendon. This injury allowed the hock to contact the ground, wearing through the skin and causing an ugly bleeding ulcer. Frank, a local in Canistota who noticed the limping, took the dog to the neighborhood veterinarian to see what could be done to repair the injury.

The tendon was very fragile, and surgery was imperative. A plaster cast was applied to prevent accidental tearing. When the cast was removed four weeks later, it was very disappointing to see the hock almost touch the floor when King bore his weight on it. Gradual improvement over the next two weeks brought the leg back to normal.

By this time, Frank and King were best of friends, and all attempts to locate the owner had failed, but Frank knew she was a black-haired woman, about 5'6" tall, who wore a blue shorty coat because King had momentarily turned and followed women of this description on several occasions on the street. After two years, the bond between Frank and King had solidified, and the two became inseparable.

One day, Frank answered a call. "I understand you have a German shepherd dog." Frank's heart sank. The caller could never prove that King was hers, and he vowed he'd never give up his best friend.

The flight from Chicago arrived in Sioux Falls at 2:45 P.M., and the taxi drove into Montrose an hour later. When Frank saw the black-haired woman, he tried to convince himself that this couldn't be happening. All she said was, "I'm the woman from Chicago." There was an instant bark from the backroom, and King came bounding out to meet his owner. Immediately, he jumped up to her, wildly wagging his tail and smiling all over. What could Frank say? The immediate recognition removed any doubt that he had hoped for.

King had flown out to Winner, South Dakota with his master and three other pheasant hunters for the weekend. He was left alone in the plane when a storm broke and buffeted the light plane. King chewed his way through the fabric side and headed for home eight hundred miles away. That was where he first met Frank.

King was flown back to Chicago where he sired "Son of King." When the pup was six months old, he joined Frank in Montrose, and stayed. Frank was paid in full.

A Short Tail

Reprinted with permission from *The Prairie Practitioners*

One Sunday afternoon, I received an urgent phone call from a pet owner. His dog had been bitten by a rattlesnake, and he would soon be brought to the clinic. The poor dog was in shock and was covered with mud and blood. I looked at the bitten area and realized that the owner had packed the area with mud. After treating her, giving her antivenom, and getting her over the shock, I began looking for the source of the blood. About one third of the dog's tail was missing. The owner casually informed me that he had cut it off. He said that with snake bite, the poison goes to the tail before it goes to the brain. By cutting off the tail, he had allowed the poison to escape! I proceeded to amputate the tail. When he picked up the dog two days later, I told him to be sure to keep the dog away from snakes, since her valuable tail was gone.

The Thief Swallows Three Carats

Submitted by R. G. MacKintosh, DVM, Yakima, Washington

A brilliantly lacquered lady, and her obviously wealthy and docile husband, glided through the waiting room and into the exam area where she demanded that her diamond-collared miniature French poodle, Cherie, be operated upon immediately.

"What is the problem?" I asked.

"She ate my ring. My diamond solitaire! It is a three-carat stone."

"Are you certain?" I asked.

And the answer was, "Yes!"

"Obviously," my diamond lady whined, "My dog needs a gastrotomy now!"

"Why don't we take an x-ray and find out for sure before we do anything as drastic as the operation, when the ring could be on the floor or behind some furniture," I cautioned. "Let's not operate unless we have to." She begrudgingly agreed.

I took Cherie to x-ray while the woman fumed at the delay. The little dog was happy and, it seemed, a little relieved to get away from the harping. The picture was developed and voilà! There it was. This dog, with his diamond-studded collar and fancy pedigree, was indeed worth a small fortune.

We were then able to confirm the location of the ring, and our calmness convinced the man, if not the lady, that the dog could safely be left at our hospital for a few days to see if nature would take its course. Cherie stayed, after her owners had been assured that we had a very good alarm system, and that she need not worry about loss of the dog. We were very patient, and the dog was released into a clean run for natural duties. The progress of the ring was followed to be sure that no intestinal blockage would interfere with nature, and the kennel man was instructed to save every stool for proper inspection. (There was a twenty in it for him, if and when recovery occurred—and it happened.)

Soap and water were applied, then the ultra-sonic cleaner and, of course, a phone call was placed to the lacquered lady, who wondered why it had taken so long. Cherie went home without a scar on her tummy, but with a bath and comb-out. The kennel man got his extra, but I have always wished that I had charged more for the services rendered.

Some doctors had stories they couldn't resist submitting. Some are heartbreaking, some are ironic, and some are humorous.

If you have a wonderful dog story, send it to Dr. Rex Puterbaugh in care of Carol Publishing Group, 120 Enterprise Avenue, Secaucus, New Jersey, 07094. It may be used for the next collection of funny dog stories.